Introduction

The chief objective of this appendix is to present, over the span of a few pages, a listing of combination chemotherapy regimens currently used in the treatment of malignant diseases (abbreviations used herein are shown in table A-1).

These regimens include, with sufficient details, drug dosages, their route, and frequency of administration (dose adjustments related to the common side effects these drugs produce are listed in a table at the end). This compendium includes the more frequently used chemotherapeutic cytotoxotic agents and the reductions that must be applied to their calculated dose in relation to some of the side effects they induce on various organs and systems.

This appendix does not contain an exhaustive presentation of all of the side effects that can possibly be caused by the recommended drugs, nor the details of therapeutic measures that can counteract or control these side effects. Also, full details on administration of these drugs are not included. It is the belief of the editor that such details cannot be entirely reduced to writing; some can be acquired only through clinical experience. For this reason, administration of the combination chemotherapy regimens presented in this appendix should be directed and carried out only by specialized physicians, medical oncologists, hematologists, or gynecologic oncologists with adequate training and experience in the field of therapy of malignant neoplasms. This appendix is intended primarily to serve these specialists as well as the trainees in the respective specialties as a useful reference for the exact dosage and sequence of administration of drugs included in relatively complex combination regimens.

The editor as well as the publisher of this book would like to caution physicians who lack adequate training in this field not to administer the regimens listed in this appendix without adequate supervision of qualified physicians. Although every effort was made to check the accuracy of the drug regimens published herein, the editor and publisher cannot take responsibility for any error that could occur in the way in which these drugs are administered resulting from their use under the direction of inexperienced physicians.

The choice of the combination chemotherapy regimens presented here followed several criteria. For malignant neoplasms in which drug regimens with curative intent exist (e.g., acute leukemias, lymphomas, germ cell tumors), as well as for advanced neoplasms in which significant prolongation of survival can be achieved by chemotherapy (e.g., breast cancer, small-cell lung cancer), all combination regimens known to have led to successful outcomes have been listed.

Conversely, for other advanced malignant tumors representing the approximately 70% of all neoplasms for which no chemotherapy that could meaningfully prolong survival has been clearly identified, the choice of combination chemotherapy regimens was somewhat arbitrary. The regimens given include some of those most commonly used as well as some that, in the opinion of the editor, are among the most effective currently (November 1990) available and have tolerable side effects.

The appendix also includes, in a section on supportive therapy, the exact formulations for antiemetic and analgesic drugs widely used in the palliation of symptoms in patients with advanced neoplasms.

This appendix does not represent an exhaustive compendium of all combination chemotherapy regimens that have ever led to favorable results in patients with advanced malignancies; rather, it includes concise listings of the most commonly used drug regimens in clinical practice that could help the practicing oncologist to prescribe a detailed and complex regimen without needing to consult the original reference.

It is hoped that this compendium of chemotherapy regimens will be useful in the daily practice of clinical oncology.

Hematologic Malignancies

Acute Myelocytic Leukemia

Regimen	Drugs	Dose/admin. rte.	Days of treatment	Frequency/ comments
Remission Induction Regimens				
DA	Daunorubicin	45 mg/m²/d I.V. bolus	1,2,3	q. 3–4 wk
	Cytosine arabinoside (ara-C)	100 mg/m²/d I.V.C.I.	1–7	1–3 times until CR
DAT	Daunorubicin	45 mg/m²/d I.V. bolus	1,2,3	q. 3–4 wk × 1–3 cyc until CR
	Cytosine arabinoside	100 mg/m²/d I.V.C.I.	1–7	
	Thioguanine	100 mg/m² p.o. q. 12 h	1–7	
MA	Mitoxantrone	12 mg/m²/d I.V. bolus	1,2,3,17,18	
	Cytosine arabinoside (ara-C)	100 mg/m²/d I.V.C.I.	1–7 & 17–21	
NOVE	Mitoxantrone (Novantrone)	10 mg/m²/d I.V. bolus	1–5	q. 3–4 wk × 2–3 cyc until CR
	Etoposide	100 mg/m²d I.V.Sh.I.	1–5	
IDAC	Idarubicin	12 mg/m²/d I.V. bolus	1–3	q. 3–4 wk × 2–3 cyc until CR
	Cytosine arabinoside	100 mg/m²/d I.V.C.I.	1–7	
L-10 MSKCC	Vincristine	1.5 mg/m² (max 2 mg) I.V. bolus	1,8,15,22,29	
(VDPM-	Prednisone	60 mg/m²/d p.o.	1–29, then D/C on d 36	
CTACy)	Doxorubicin	20 mg/m² I.V. bolus	17,18,19	
	Methotrexate	15 mg/m² I.V. bolus	42–46; 78–82; 114–118	
		6.25 mg/m² i. thec, or Omaya reserv	2,5,16,19,30,33, 55,58,88,92,95	
	Cytosine arabinoside (ara-c)	30 mg/kg I.V. 3-h inf q. 12 h	56–63;92–98; 128–134	
	Thioguanine	2.5 mg/kg p.o. q. 12 h	56–63;92–98; 128–134	
	Asparaginase	200 IU/kg I.V. 1-h inf	135–144	
	Cyclophosphamide	1,200 mg/m² 2-h inf	146	
Consolidation Regimens				
HiC-D	Cytosine arabinoside (high-dose)	3 gm/m² q. 12 h I.V. 3-h inf	1–6	Admin c̄ antiemetics, steroid ophthalmic drops, KCL
	Daunorubicin	30 mg/m² I.V. bolus	7,8	
HiC-AMSA	Cytosine arabinoside	3 gm/m² q. 12 h I.V. 3-h inf	1–5	This and previous regimen can also be used for reinduction of remissions after DA or DAT regimen
	M-AMSA	100 mg/m² I.V.Sh.I.	1–5	
D/DA	Doxorubicin (Adriamycin) *or*	45 mg/m²/d I.V. bolus	1	q. 4 wk × 2
	Daunorubicin	55 mg/m²/d I.V. bolus	1	
	Cytosine arabinoside	200 mg/m²/d I.V.C.I.	1–5	
Maintenance Regimens				
CT	Cytosine arabinoside	100 mg/m² s.c. q. 12 h	1–5	q. 4 wk × 12
	Thioguanine	50 mg/m² p.o. q. 12 h	1–5	
TC	Thioguanine	40 mg/m² p.o. q. 12 h	1–4	q. wk × 26
	Cytosine arabinoside	60 mg/m² s.c.	5	

Acute Lymphocytic Leukemia

Regimen	Drugs/ procedures	Dose & admin. rte.	Days of treatment	Frequency & comments
Induction Regimens				
1. *For Favorable Childhood ALL (L-1)*				
PVD (M-CRT)	Prednisone	40 mg/m^2/d p.o.	1–28, then taper down; D/C on d 36	
	Vincristine	1.5 mg/m^2/d (to max 2 mg) I.V. bolus	1,8,15,22	
	Daunorubicin	45 mg/m^2/d I.V. bolus	1,8,15,22 *or* 1,2,3	
	Methotrexate	12 mg/m^2 (max 15 mg) i. thec.	30,32,37,39,44 or early if CNS is involved	
	Cranial irradiation	15 fractions to total	29–33	
		2,400 cGy for >2 yr old	36–40	
		2,000 cGy for 1–2 yr old	43–47	
		1,500 cGy for <1 yr old		
2. *For Poor-Prognosis Childhood ALL (L-1), Adult ALL (L-2), and Burkitt's-like ALL (L-3)*				
CALBG (VDPAM)	Vincristine	1.4 mg/m^2 (max 2 mg) I.V. bolus	1,8,15	
	Daunorubicin	45 mg/m^2/d I.V. bolus	1,2,3	
	Prednisone	40 mg/m^2/d p.o.	1–22, then taper down; D/C on d 29	
	Asparaginase	500 IU/kg/d (max 10,000) I.V. 1-h inf	22–31	
	Methotrexate	6.25 mg/m^2 i.thec. or Omaya reserv	8,15,22,29	The admin in CSF should continue 2 × after CSF becomes normal in case of CNS leukemia
Consolidation or Remission Reinduction Regimen				
H.DAC ASNase	Cytosine arabinoside (ara-C)	3 gm/m^2 I.V. 3-h inf q. 12 h	1,2,8,9	
	Asparaginase	6,000 IU/m^2 3 h after last ara-C dose	2 & 9	
AVDP	Asparaginase	15,000 IU/m^2 I.V.Sh.I.	1–5;8–12;15–19,22–26.	
	Vincristine	2 mg/m^2 (max 2 mg) I.V. bolus	8,15,22	
	Daunorubicin	30–60 mg/m^2 I.V. bolus	8,15,22	
	Prednisone	40 mg/m^2 p.o. q.d.	8–12;15–19;22–26	
Maintenance Regimens				
MVP Met	6-Mercaptopurine	50 mg/m^2 p.o.	q.d. × 10 wk	q. 12 wk × 3
	Methotrexate	15 mg/m^2 p.o.	q.d. on day 1 of wk 1–10	
		and		
		12 mg/m^2 (max 15 mg) i. thec. or Omaya reserv	q.d. on d 1 of wk 11 & 12	
	Prednisone	40 mg/m^2 p.o.	q.d. of wk 11 & 12	
	Vincristine	1.5 mg/m^2 (max 2 mg)	q.d. on d 1 of wk 11 & 12	

Chronic Lymphocytic Leukemia

Regimen	Drugs	Dose & admin. rte.	Days of treatment	Frequency & comments
ChP	Chlorambucil	0.4–0.6 mg/kg p.o.	1	q. 3–4 wk
	Prednisone	60 mg/m^2 p.o. q.d.	1–4	until WBC nadir is 5,000/μl
CVP	Cyclophosphamide	300 mg/m^2 p.o. q.d.	1–5	q. 4 wk until WBC
		or 1,000 mg/m^2 I.V.	1	nadir is 3,000/μl or
	Vincristine	1 mg/m^2	1	q. 4 wk × 6, then q.
		I.V. bolus	1	12 wk × 6
	Prednisone	40 mg/m^2 p.o.	1–5	
CHOP	Cyclophosphamide	300 mg/m^2 p.o.	1–5	q. 4 wk × 6,
	Adriamycin (hydroxydaunorubicin)	25 mg/m^2 I.V. bolus	1	then q. 12 wk × 6 Recommended
	Vincristine (Oncovin)	1 mg/m^2 I.V. bolus	1	only for pts in
	Prednisone	40 mg/m^2 p.o.	1–5	stage C (Binet) or stages III & IV (Rai)
Fludarabine	Fludarabine	20 mg/m^2 I.V.	1–5	q. 4 wk until WBC nadir is 3000/μl or progression occurs

Hairy Cell Leukemia

Regimen	Drugs	Dose & admin. rte.	Days of treatment	Frequency & comments
INF	Alpha 2a or b interferon	3 × 10^6 U/d s.c. or I.M.	t.i.w.	q. wk × 26–52
PENT	2′-Deoxycoformicin (Pentostatin)	4 mg/m^2 I.V.	q. wk × 3	q. 8 wk × 6

Multiple Myeloma

Regimen	Drugs	Dose & admin. rte.	Days of treatment	Frequency & comments
VMCP	Vincristine	1 mg/m^2 (max 2 mg) I.V. bolus	1	q. 21 d
	Melphalan	5 mg/m^2/d p.o.	1–4	
	Cyclophosphamide	100 mg/m^2/d p.o.	1–4	
	Prednisone	40 mg/m^2/d p.o.	1–4	
MP	Melphalan	0.15 mg/kg/d p.o., then when CBC rises, 0.05 mg/kg/d p.o.	1–7 daily	Continuously
	Prednisone	0.8 mg/kg/d p.o. (max 100 mg/d)	1–14, then taper down for 6 wk	

Regimen	Drugs	Dose & admin. rte.	Days of treatment	Frequency & comments
VMCP-VCAP	Vincristine	1 mg/m^2 (max 2 mg) I.V. bolus	1 & 22	q. 42 d
	Melphalan	5 mg/m^2/d p.o.	1–4	
	Cyclophosphamide	100 mg/m^2/d p.o.	1–4;22–25	
	Prednisone	60 mg/m^2/d p.o.	1–4;22–25	
	Doxorubicin (Adriamycin)	25 mg/m^2 I.V. bolus	22	
M2	Melphalan	0.25 mg/kg/d p.o.	1–4	q. 28 d
	Prednisone	1 mg/kg/d p.o.	1–7	
	Vincristine	0.03 mg/kg I.V. bolus	1	
	Carmustine	1 mg/kg I.V.Sh.I.	1	
	Cyclophosphamide	10 mg/kg I.V.Sh.I.	1	
BCP	Carmustine (BCNU)	75 mg/m^2 I.V.Sh.I.	1	q. 28 d
	Cyclophosphamide	400 mg/m^2 I.V.Sh.I.	1	
	Prednisone	75 mg. p.o.	1–7	
VAD	Vincristine	0.4 mg/d (mixed in same I.V. solution with ADR) I.V.C.I. through central vein indwelling cath	1–4	q. 28 d
	Doxorubicin (Adriamycin)	9 mg/m^2		
	Dexamethasone	40 mg p.o.	1–4 9–12 17–20	
VBAP	Vincristine	2 mg I.V. bolus	1	q. 3–4 wk
	Carmustine (BCNU)	30 mg/m^2 I.V.Sh.I.	1	
	Doxorubicin (Adriamycin)	30 mg/m^2 I.V. bolus	1	
	Prednisone	20 mg t.i.d. p.o.	1–5	

DOSE ADJUSTMENTS—MULTIPLE MYELOMA

1. For all multiple myeloma combination chemotherapy regimens, dose attenuations due to bone marrow suppression are recommended for the following drugs: melphalan, cyclophosphamide, Adriamycin, and carmustine:

Granulocytes/μl	Platelets/μl	Doses administered
≥3,000	130,000	Full doses
2,000–2,990	100,000–129,000	50% of calc dose
1,500–2,000	75,000–99,990	25% of calc dose
<1,500	<75,000	Hold therapy & reevaluate within 1 wk × 2

2. Vincristine dose should be adjusted in relation to the development of peripheral neuropathy as follows:

—Dose should be reduced by 50% in case of markedly diminished deep tendon reflexes (DTRs) or persistent constipation despite adequate administration of catharics.

—Administration should be withheld if patient starts walking with a shuffling gait, if DTRs are absent, or if paralytic ileus develops.

3. Vincristine dose should also be reduced when serum direct bilirubin is rising:

—by 25% for >1.2 ≤1.5 mg/dl direct bilirubin

—by 50% for <2.5 ≤1.5 mg/dl

—by 75% for >2.5 mg/dl

Hodgkin's Disease

Regimen	Drugs	Dose & admin. rte.	Days of treatment	Frequency & comments
MOPP	Mechlorethamine (HN2) (Mustargen)	6 mg/m^2 I.V. bolus in a running inf	1 & 8	q. 28 d × 6
	Vincristine (Oncovin)	1.4 mg/m^2 I.V. bolus (max 2 mg)	1 & 8	
	Procarbazine	100 mg/m^2 p.o.	1–14	Diet without ripe cheese, avocado, nuts
	Prednisone	40 mg/m^2 p.o.	1–14	Only on 1st & 4th cyc
C-MOPP (same as MOPP but HN2 replaced by C if nausea and vomiting are intolerable)	Cyclophosphanide	650 mg/m^2 I.V.Sh.I.	1 & 8	
MVPP (same as MOPP but O replaced by V)	Vinblastine	6 mg/m^2 I.V. bolus	1 & 8	
ABVD	Doxorubicin (Adriamycin)	25 mg/m^2 I.V. bolus	1 & 15	q. 28 d × 6
	Bleomycin	2 U/d s.c.	4–10;18–24	
	Vinblastine	6 mg/m^2 I.V. bolus (max 10 mg)	1 & 15	
	Dacarbazine	250 mg/m^2 I.V.Sh.I. (200 cc D5%/W)	1 & 15	
MOPP/ABVD	MOPP		1–28	q. 56 d × 3
	ABVD		29–56	
MOPP/ABV Hybrid	Mechlorethamine (Mustargen)	6 mg/m^2 I.V. in a running inf	1	q. 28 d × 6
	Vincristine (Oncovin)	1.4 mg/m^2 I.V. bolus (max 2 mg)	1	
	Procarbazine	100 mg/m^2/d p.o.	1–7	Same diet restrictions
	Prednisone	40 mg/m^2/d p.o.	1–14	
	Doxorubicin (Adriamycin)	35 mg/m^2/d I.V. bolus	8	
	Bleomycin	10 U/m^2 I.V. inf after test dose	8	Should be preceded by hydrocortisone 100 mg I.V.
	Vinblastine	6 mg/m^2 I.V. bolus	8	
CVPD	Lomustine (CCNU)	75 mg/m^2 p.o.	1	q. 28 d
	Vinblastine	4 mg/m^2 I.V. bolus	1 & 8	
	Procarbazine	100 mg/m^2 p.o.	1–14	Same diet restrictions
	Prednisone	30 mg/m^{2}p.o.	1–14	Only on 1st & 4th cyc
ACOPP (used in children)	Doxorubicin (Adriamycin)	60 mg/m^2 I.V. bolus	1	q. 42 d × 6
	Cyclophosphamide	300 mg/m^2 I.V.Sh.I.	14 & 20	
	Vincristine (Oncovin)	1.5 mg/m^2 (max 2 mg) I.V. bolus	14 & 20	
	Procarbazine	100 mg/m^2 p.o.	14–20	
	Prednisone	40 mg/m^2 p.o.	1–27 in cyc 1 & 4; 14–27 in cyc 2,3,5 & 6	

Regimen	Drugs	Dose & admin. rte.	Days of treatment	Frequency & comments
Salvage Regimens				
CAV	Lomustine (CCNU)	100 mg/m^2 p.o.	1	q. 42 d × 6
	Melphalan (Alkeran)	6 mg/m^2 p.o.	1–4;22–26	
	Vinblastine	4 mg/m^2 I.V. bolus	1 & 22	
CEM	Lomustine (CCNU)	120 mg/m^2 p.o.	1	q. 42 d
	Etoposide	100 mg/m^2 I.V.Sh.I. *or* 200 mg/m^2 p.o.	1,2,3, & 22,23, 24 1,2,3 and 22,23,24	
	Methotrexate	200 mg/m^2 I.V.Sh.I.	1 & 22	
	Leucovorin	25 mg p.o. q. 6 h × 8	2,3, & 23, 24	

Non-Hodgkin's Lymphoma

Regimen	Drugs	Dose (mg/m^2) & admin. rte.	Days of treatment	Frequency & comments
C-MOPP	Cyclophosphamide	650 I.V.	1 & 8	q. 28 d × 6–12 cyc
	Vincristine (Oncovin)	1.4 I.V. (max 2 mg)	1 & 8	
	Procarbazine	100 p.o.	1–14	
	Prednisone	40 p.o.	1–14	
CHOP	Cyclophosphamide	750 I.V.	1	q. 21 d × 8–10 cyc (max doxorubicin dose 450 mg/m^2; for >300 mg/m^2 total dose, monitor ventric ejec fraction)
	Doxorubicin (hydroxydaunomycin)	50 I.V.	1	
	Vincristine (Oncovin)	1.4 I.V. (max 2 mg)	1 & 5	
	Prednisone	100 p.o.	1–5	
CHOP-Bleo	Cyclophosphamide	750 I.V.	1	q. 21 d × 8 (same restrictions as above for doxorubicin)
	Doxorubicin (hydroxydaunomycin)	50 I.V.	1	
	Vincristine (Oncovin)	1.4 I.V. (max 2 mg)	1	
	Prednisone	100 p.o.	1–5	
	Bleomycin	4 I.V.	1	
BCVP	Carmustine (BCNU)	60 I.V.	1	q. 21 d × 6–12 cyc
	Cyclophosphamide	1,000 I.V.	1	
	Vincristine (Oncovin)	1.4 I.V. (max 2 mg)	1	
	Prednisone	100 p.o.	1 & 15	
BACOP	Bleomycin	5 I.V.	15 & 21	q. 28 d × 5–10 cyc
	Doxorubicin (Adriamycin)	25 I.V.	1 & 8	
	Cyclophosphamide	650 I.V.	1 & 8	
	Vincristine (Oncovin)	1.4 I.V. (max 2 mg)	1 & 8	
	Prednisone	60 p.o.	15–28	
COMLA	Cyclophosphamide	1,500 I.V.	1	q. 12 wk × 3
	Vincristine (Oncovin)	1.5 I.V. (max 2 mg)	1,8 & 15	
	Methotrexate	120 I.V.	22, then weekly × 7	
	Leucovorin	15 p.o. q. 6 h × 8	23,24 (24 h after MTX) then weekly × 7	
	Cytosine arabinoside	300 I.V.	22, then weekly × 7	

Regimen	Drugs	Dose (mg/m^2) & admin. rte.	Days of treatment	Frequency & comments
m-BACOD	Methotrexate	200 I.V.	8 & 15	q. 21–28 d × 6–10 cyc
	Leucovorin	15 p.o. q. 6 h × 8	9,10; 16,17 (start 24 h after beginning MTX inf)	
	Bleomycin	4 I.V.	1	
	Doxorubicin (Adriamycin)	45 I.V.	1	
	Cyclophosphamide	600 I.V.	1	
	Vincristine (Oncovin)	1.0 I.V. (max 2 mg)	1	
	Dexamethasone	6 p.o.	1–5	
ProMACE	Prednisone	60 p.o.	1–14	q. 28 d × 6–10 cyc
	Methotrexate	1,500 I.V.	14	
	Leucovorin	15 p.o. q. 6 h × 8	15,16	
	Doxorubicin (Adriamycin)	25 I.V.	1 & 8	
	Cyclophosphamide	650 I.V.	1 & 8	
	Etoposide	120 I.V.	1 & 8	
ProMace-MOPP (flexi-therapy)	ProMace		1–14	q. 56 d × 6
	Standard MOPP		29–43	
ACOMLA	Doxorubicin (Adriamycin)	40 I.V.	1	q. 3 mo × 3
	Cyclophosphamide	1,000 I.V.	1	
	Vincristine (Oncovin)	2 I.V. (total)	1,8,15	
	Methotrexate	120 I.V.	22,29,36,43,50, 57,64,71	
	Leucovorin	25 p.o. (total)	24 h after MTX, q. 6 h × 6	
	Cytosine arabinoside (ara-C)	300 I.V.	1 hr after MTX on same days	
Pro-MACE (S Mtx)	Prednisone	60 p.o.	1–14	q. 21 d × 6–12 cyc
CYTABOM	Doxorubicin (Adriamycin)	25 I.V. bolus	1	
	Cyclophosphamide	650 I.V.Sh.I.	1	
	Etoposide	120 I.V.Sh.I.	1	
	Cytarabine	300 I.V.	8	
	Bleomycin	5 I.V.	8	
	Methotrexate	120 I.V.	8	
	Leucovorin	25 p.o. (total)	9 q. 6 h × 8 (24 h after MTX)	
COP-BLAM-III	Cyclophosphamide	350 I.V. (escalate to 500)	1 & 22	q. 6 wk × 6–8 cyc
	Vincristine (Oncovin)	1 I.V.C.I.	1–2	
		1.4 (max 2) I.V. bolus	22	
	Prednisone	40 p.o. q.d.	1–5; 22–27	
	Bleomycin	7.5 I.V. bolus *and*	1 & 22	
		7.5/d I.V.C.I.	1–5	
	Doxorubicin (Adriamycin)	35 I.V. bolus (escalate to 50)	1 & 22	
	Procarbazine (Matulane)	100 p.o	1–5; 22–27	

Regimen	Drugs	Dose (mg/m^2) & admin. rte.	Days of treatment	Frequency & comments
MACOP-B	Methotrexate	400 I.V.Sh.I. (hydration, alkalization of urine)	1 of wk 2,6,10	
	Doxorubicin (Adriamycin)	50 I.V. bolus	1 of wk 1,3,5,7,9,11	
	Cyclophosphamide	350 I.V.Sh.I.	1 of wk 1,3,5,7,9,11	
	Vincristine (Oncovin)	1.4 I.V. bolus	1 of wk 2,4,6,8,10,12	
	Bleomycin	10 U I.V. bolus	1 of wk 4,8,12	
	Prednisone	45 p.o.	q.d.; dose tapered over last 15 d	
	Co-trimoxazole	1 double-strength tab p.o.	b.i.d. throughout cyc	
VACOP-B	Etoposide (VP-16)	50 I.V.Sh.I.	1 of wk 3,7,11	
		100 p.o.	2,3 of wk 3,7,11	
	Doxorubicin (Adriamycin)	50 I.V. bolus	1 of wk 1,3,5,7,9,11	
	Cyclophosphamide	350 I.V.Sh.I.	1 of wk 1,3,5,7,9,11	
	Vincristine (Oncovin)	1.2 I.V. bolus	1 of wk 2,4,6,8,10,12	
	Bleomycin	10 I.V. bolus	1 of wk 2,4,6,8,10,12	
	Prednisone	45 p.o.	q.d. × 1 wk, then q.o.d. × 11 wk	
	Ketoconazole	200 p.o.	daily × 1 wk, then q.o.d. × 11 wk	
	Cimetidine	600 p.o.	b.i.d. × 1 wk, then q.o.d. × 11 wk	
	Co-trimoxazole	1 double-strength tab p.o.	b.i.d. throughout cyc	
MINE	MESNA (uroprotector)	1.33 g/m^2/d I.V.C.I.	1–4	
			1–4 q. 28 d × 6 cyc	
	Ifosfamide	1.33 g/m^2/d I.V.C.I.	1–3	
	Mitoxantrone (Novantrone)	8 I.V. bolus	1	
	Etoposide	65 I.V.Sh.I.	1–3	
IMVP-16	Ifosfamide	4g/m^2/d I.V.C.I.	1	q. 21–28 d × 6–8 cyc
	MESNA	4g/m^2/d I.V.C.I.	1 & 2	
	Etoposide (VP-16)	100 I.V.	1–3	
LSA2-L2 (pediatric cases; induction and consolidation phase)	Cyclophosphamide	1,200 I.V. bolus	1	
	Vincristine	1.5 (max) I.V. bolus	3,10,17,24	
	Prednisone	60 p.o. in 3 divided doses	3–31	
	Methotrexate	6.25 i.thec.	5,27,30,85,88	
	Daunorubicin	60 I.V. bolus	12,13	
	XRT (concomitantly to bulky disease)			
	Cytosine arabinoside	150 I.V. bolus	36–40; 43–47	
	Thioguanine	75 p.o. (8–12 h after cytosine arabinoside)	36–40; 43–47	
	Asparaginase	6,000 U/m^2	70–81	
	Carmustine	60 I.V. inf over 1 h	90	

Regimen	Drugs	Dose (mg/m^2) & admin. rte.	Days of treatment	Frequency & comments
LSA2-L2 (maintenance phase; start on day 94 of induction and consolidation phase)	Thioguanine	300 p.o.	1–4	q. 10 wk for total of 2–3 yr
	Cyclophosphamide	600 I.V.	5	
	Hydroxyurea	500 p.o.	15–18	
	Daunorubicin	45 I.V. bolus	19	
	Methotrexate	10 p.o.	30–33	
	Carmustine	60 I.V. (1-hr inf)	34	
	Cytosine arabinoside	150 I.V. bolus	44–47	
	Vincristine	1.5 (max 2) I.V. bolus	48	
	Methotrexate	6.25 i.thec.	58 & 61	
COMP (pediatric cases; induction phase)	Cyclophosphamide	1,200 I.V. 250 ml D5%/W	1	
	Vincristine (Oncovin)	2 (max) I.V. push	3,10,17,24	
	Methorexate	300 I.V. (60% of dose as I.V. push and 40% as 4-h inf in D5%/W)	12	
	Methotrexate	6.25 i.thec.	5,31,34	
	Prednisone	60 (max) p.o. q.d. in 4 divided doses	3–30	
COMP (maintenance phase; starts 7–21 d after last i.thec. MTX of induction)	Cyclophosphamide	1,000 I.V. inf in 250 ml D5%/W	1	q. 28 d × 18 mo
	Vincristine (Oncovin)	1.5 (max 2) I.V. bolus	1 & 14	
	Methotrexate	6.25 i.thec.	29 (1 of 2nd cycle)	
	Methotrexate	300 I.V. (60% of dose as I.V. push and 40% as 4-h inf in D5%/W	15	
	Prednisone	60 (max) p.o. q.d.	29 (1 of 2nd cyc) to 33 (5 of 2nd cyc)	
ACE	Cytosine arabinoside (ara-C)	150–300 24 h I.V.C.I.	1 & 8	q. 28 d × 4–6 cyc
	Cisplatin	80 I.V.Sh.I. with hydration, mannitol, antiemetics	1	
	Etoposide	100 I.V.Sh.I. *or* 200 p.o.	1 & 8	
HEIM	Hydroxyurea	1 g/m^2 p.o. q. 6 h	1 & 2	q. 21 d × 6 cyc
	Etoposide	80 I.V.Sh.I. then 160 p.o.	4 & 5 6	
	Ifosfamide	3 g/m^2 I.V.C.I.	4	
	MESNA	3 g/m^2 I.V.C.I.	4 & 5	

DOSE ADJUSTMENTS—ALL LYMPHOMA REGIMENS (HODGKIN'S DISEASE AND NON-HODGKIN'S LYMPHOMAS)

The following general recommendations can be made:

1. In case of bone marrow suppression reflected by low granulocyte and platelet counts, the dosage of these drugs should be decreased: cyclophosphamide, mechlorethamine, procarbazine, doxorubicin, carmustine, lomustine, cytosine arabinoside, methotrexate, etoposide, ifosfamide, dacarbazine, and vinblastine.

Granulocytes/µl	Platelets/µl	Doses administered
>3,000	130,000	Full doses
3,000–2,990	100,000–129,000	75% of calc dose
1,500–1,990	75,000–99,000	50% of calc dose
<1,500	75,000	Hold therapy

2. Vinblastine, vincristine, and doxorubicin should also be adjusted for cholestasis as follows:

Direct bilirubin level	Doses administered
<1.2 mg	Full dose
1.2–1.5	75% of calc dose
1.5–2.5	50% of calc dose
>2.5	Hold therapy

3. Bleomycin should not be administered beyond a total dose of 150 U/m^2 or whenever a drop by >20% of patient's diffusion capacity is noted or "interstitial streaking" develops on plain chest x-ray not explained by other pathologic process.

4. Vincristine and vinblastine doses should be decreased by 50% if DTRs are diminished or severe constipation develops. The drug should be discontinued when DTRs are completely suppressed.

Malignant Tumors of the Brain

Regimen	Drugs	Dose & admin. rte.	Days of treatment	Frequency & comments
Glioblastoma Multiforme				
BCNU-XRT	Carmustine (BCNU)	100 mg/m^2 I.V. 1-h inf *or* 80 mg/m^2 I.V. 1-h inf	1,2 1,2,3	q. 6–8 wk × 6–10 cyc (1st cyc starts at same time as XRT & dexamethasone)
CCNU-XRT	Lomustine (CCNU)	120 mg/m^2 p.o. q.d.	1,2	q. 6 wk × 6–10 cyc (1st cyc starts at same time as XRT & dexamethasone)
BP-XRT	Lomustine (BCNU) Cisplatin (Platinol)	100 mg/m^2 I.V. 1-h inf 80 mg/m^2 I.V. with mannitol, hydration, antiemetics	1 1,22	q. 6 wk × 6 cyc (1st cyc starts at same time as XRT & dexamethasone)
Meduloblastoma				
CVP	Lomustine (CCNU) Vincristine Cisplatin (Platinol)	75 mg/m^2 p.o. 1.5 mg/m^2 (max 2 mg) I.V. 75 mg/m^2 I.V. in short NS inf with hydration, antiemetics, mannitiol	1 1,8,15,22 29,36,43,50 1,22	q. 42 × 8 cyc (except for vincristine, to be D/C after 8 wk) (1st cyc accompanies XRT & dexamthasone)

DOSE ADJUSTMENTS—MALIGNANT TUMORS OF THE BRAIN

1. For carmustine and lomustine, doses are related to the degree of bone marrow suppression:

Granulocytes/µl	Platelets/µl	Dose administered
≥3,000	≥130,000	Full dose
2,000–2,990	100,000–129,000	75% of calc dose
1,500–1,990	75,000–99,000	50% of calc dose
<1,500	<75,000	Hold therapy

2. For vincristine, dose should be decreased by 50% if deep tendon reflexes are decreased, if severe constipation persists, or serum direct bilirubin is 1.5–2.5 mg/dl. The drug should be withheld when DTRs are absent or serum direct bilirubin is >2.5 mg/dl.
3. Administration of cisplatin should be postponed when serum creatinine is 1.5 mg/dl or creatinine clearance is <60 ml/hr.

Head and Neck Cancer

For patients with unresectable or recurrent or metastatic lesions, no known standard chemotherapy regimens can prolong survival significantly. Regimens listed below are among those suggested for patients not eligible for clinical trials.

Regimen	Drugs	Dosage (mg/m^2) & admin. rte.	Days of treatment	Frequency & comments
PF	Cisplatin (Platinol)	100 I.V.Sh.I. with mannitol, I.V. hydration, antiemetics	1	q. 3 wk × 10–12 cyc
		or		
		20 I.V. bolus c̄ same support	1–5	
	5-Fluorouracil	1,000/24 h. I.V.C.I.	1–5 *or* 2–6	
MBP	Methotrexate	40 I.M.	1 & 15	q. 3 wk × 6
	Bleomycin	10 (total dose) I.M.	1 & 15	
	Cisplatin (Platinol)	50 I.V. bolus c̄ supp. meas.	day 4	
PBML	Cisplatin (Platinol)	20 I.V. bolus c̄ supp. meas.	1–6	q. 3 wk × 4–6 cyc
	Bleomycin	10 I.V. 24-h inf	3–7	
	Methotrexate (high-dose)	240–700 I.V. Inf in D5%/½ NS	1	
	Leucovorin	50 I.V.	2	
		15 p.o.	q. 6 hr days 2,3,4	
MLF	Methotrexate	240 I.V. in 500 ml NS over 4 h	1	q. 3 wk
	Leucovorin	50 I.V. in 50 ml D5%/½ NS over 2 h	2 (24 h after MTX is started)	
		15 p.o.	q. 6 h days 2, 3	
	5-Fluorouracil	600 I.V. bolus 1 h after leucovorin is started	2	
COB	Cisplatin	100 I.V. c̄ supp. meas.	1	q. 21 d × 6 cyc
	Vincristine (Oncovin)	1 I.V.	1 & 5	
	Bleomycin	30/day I.V.C.I.	2–5	Only in first 3 cyc
MBC	Methotrexate	40 I.V. bolus or I.M.	1 & 15	q. 21 d × 3
	Bleomycin	10 I.V. or I.M.	1,8,15	
	Cisplatin	50 I.V. c̄ supp. meas.	4	
BPVM	Bleomycin	5 U/m^2/24 h I.V.C.I. in 1,000 ml NS alone or admixed c̄ DDP	1–5	× 28 d × 6 cyc
	Cisplatin (Platinol)	20 I.V. push *or* admixed c̄ BLM in 1,000 ml NS (hydration, mannitol, antiemetics)	1–5	
	Vinblastine	6 I.V. bolus	1	
	or			
	Etoposide (VP-16)	50 I.V.Sh.I.	1,3,5	
	Methotrexate	40 I.V. bolus (before DDP)	1	

Lung Cancer

Small-Cell Lung Cancer

Regimen	Drugs	Dosage (mg/m^2) & admin. rte.	Days of treatment	Frequency & comments
CAV	Cyclophosphamide	1,000 I.V.Sh.I.	1	q. 3 wk × 6
	Doxorubicin (Adriamycin)	50 I.V. bolus	1	
	Vincristine	1.4 (max 2) I.V. bolus	1	
CAE	Cyclophosphamide	1,000 I.V.Sh.I.	1	q. 3 wk × 6
	Doxorubicin (Adriamycin)	50 I.V. bolus	1	
	Etoposide	50 I.V.Sh.I.	1–4	
		or		
		100 p.o.	1–4	
EP	Etoposide	50 I.V.Sh.I.	1–5	q. 3 wk × 4
		or		
		100 I.V.Sh.I.	1,3,5	
	Cisplatin (Platinol)	75–100 I.V.Sh.I. with mannitol, hydration, antiemetics	1	
EC	Etoposide	100 I.V.Sh.I.	1,2,3	q. 4 wk × 4
	Carboplatin	300 I.V.Sh.I.	1	
CAVEP (MSKCC)	Cyclophosphamide	1,200 I.V.Sh.I.	1	q. 4–5 wk × 4 cyc
	Doxorubicin (Adriamycin)	50 I.V. bolus	1	
	Vincristine	1.4 (max 2) I.V. bolus	1	
	Etoposide	120 I.V.Sh.I.	18,20,22	
	Cisplatin (Platinol)	60 I.V.Sh.I. c̄ antiemetics & mannitol	15	
CAVEP (NCI)	Cyclophosphamide	1,000 I.V.Sh.I.	1	q. 6 wk × 6
	Doxorubicin (Adriamycin)	50 I.V. bolus	1	
	Vincristine	1.4 (max 2) I.V. bolus	1	
	Etoposide	100 I.V.Sh.I.	22,23,24	
	Cisplatin (Platinol)	25 I.V.Sh.I. c̄ AE & M	22,23,24	
M-CAVEP	Cisplatin (Platinol)	50 I.V.Sh.I. c̄ AE & M	1,8	
	Etoposide	50 I.V.Sh.I.	1,2,3	
	Vincristine	1.4 (max 2) I.V. bolus	8	
	Cyclophosphamide	450 I.V.Sh.I.	15	
	Doxorubicin (Adriamycin)	50 I.V. bolus	15	
	Methotrexate	200 I.V.Sh.I.	22	
	Leucovorin	25 p.o. (total) q. 6 h × 8	23, 24	

Nonsmall-Cell Lung Cancer

In nonsmall-cell lung cancer, no known standard chemotherapy regimens can prolong survival significantly. Some suggested regimens for patients not eligible for clinical trials are listed below.

Regimen	Drugs	Dose (mg/m^2) & admin. rte.	Days of treatment	Frequency & comments
CAP	Cyclosphosphamide	500 I.V.Sh.I.	1	q. 3 wk × 6
	Doxorubicin (Adriamycin)	50 I.V. bolus	1	
	Cisplatin (Platinol)	80 I.V. NS Sh.I. with I.V. hydration, mannitol, antiemetics	1	
MVP	Mitomycin-C	10 I.V. bolus	1	q. 8 wk × 3
	Vinblastine	6 I.V. bolus	1,15,29,43	
	Cisplatin (Platinol)	100 I.V. as above	1 & 29	
EP	Etoposide	125 I.V.	1	
		125 I.V.	2,3	
		or		
		250 p.o.	2,3	
	Cisplatin	60 I.V.	1	
		or		
		20 I.V. with I.V. hydration, mannitol, antiemetics	1,2,3	
EC	Etoposide	100 I.V.	1	
		200 p.o.	2,3	
	Carboplatin	200 I.V.	1	
MEP	Mitomycin-C	10 I.V. bolus	1	q. 6 wk × 3
	Etoposide	120 I.V.Sh.I.	1 & 22	
	Cisplatin (Platinol)	80 I.V. c̄ supp. meas.	1 & 22	
MEP (5d)	Mitomycin-C	10 I.V. bolus	1	q. 8 wk × 3
	Etoposide	50 I.V.Sh.I. NS	1–5; 29–33	
	Cisplatin (Platinol)	20 I.V.Sh.I. NS c̄ supp. meas.	1–5; 29–33	
MACC	Methotrexate	40 I.V. bolus	1	q. 3 wk × 6–10 cyc
	Doxorubicin (Adriamycin)	40 I.V. bolus	1	
	Cyclosphosphamide	400 I.V.Sh.I.	1	
	Lomustine (CCNU)	30 p.o.	1	
COB	Cisplatin	100 I.V. c̄ supp. meas.	1	q. 21 d × 6
	Vincristine (Oncovin)	1 I.V.	1 & 5	
	Bleomycin	30/day I.V.C.I.	2–5	Only in the first 3 cyc
MBC	Methotrexate	40 I.V. bolus or I.M.	1 & 15	q. 21 d
	Bleomycin	10 I.V. or I.M.	1,8,15	
	Cisplatin	50 I.V. c̄ supp. meas.	4	
BPVM	Bleomycin	5 U/m^2/24 h I.V.C.I. in 1,000 ml NS alone or admixed c̄ DDP	1–5	q. 21–28 d × 5–6 cyc
	Cisplatin (Platinol)	20 I.V. push or admixed c̄ BLM in 1,000 ml NS (hydration, mannitol, antiemetics)	1–5	
	Vinblastine	6 I.V. bolus	1	q. 28 d × 6
	or			
	Etoposide	50 I.V.Sh.I.	1,3,5	
	Methotrexate	40 I.V. bolus (before DDP)	1	

Digestive System Malignancies

Esophageal Carcinoma

For recurrent or metastatic squamous cell carcinoma of the esophagus, the regimens below can be administered to patients who are not eligible for clinical trials.

For unresectable squamous cell carcinoma of the esophagus, combined modality therapy is used, with XRT given 5 days/wk (180–200 cGy/day) up to a total of 6,000–6,500 cGy; combination chemotherapy is administered every 3 wk, usually alternating chemotherapy agents as shown below.

Regimen	Drugs	Dose (mg/m^2) & admin. rte.	Days of treatment	Frequency & comments
PF	Cisplatin (Platinol)	100 I.V. NS Sh.I. or 24-h inf	1	c̄ supp. meas.
	5-Fluorouracil	1,000 I.V. D5%/½ NS I.V.C.I.	2–4	
MF	Mitomycin-C	10 I.V. bolus	22	
	5-Fluorouracil	1,000 I.V. D5%/½ NS	23–26	
MLF	Methotrexate	200 I.V.Sh.I.	43	
	Leucovorin	50 I.V. 2-h inf	44 (24 h after start of MTX)	
		then 15 p.o. q. 6 h × 8	44,45	
	5-Fluorouracil	500 I.V. bolus 1 h (after LCV is started)	44	

For recurrent or metastatic adenocarcinoma of the esophagus, regimens administered to patients with advanced gastric carcinoma (see below) can be used in patients not eligible for investigational protocols.

Gastric Carcinoma (Advanced Unresectable or Metastatic)

Regimen	Drugs	Dose (mg/m^2) & admin. rte.	Days of treatment	Frequency & comments
FAM	5-Fluourouracil	600 I.V. bolus	1,8,29,36	q. 56 d × 6
	Doxorubicin (Adriamycin)	30 I.V. bolus	1,29	
	Mitomycin-C	10 I.V. bolus	1	
APE(EAP)	Doxorubicin (Adriamycin)	20 I.V. bolus	1 & 7	q. 3–4 wk × 6
	Cisplatin (Platinol)	40 I.V. bolus c̄ supp. meas.	2 & 8	
	Etoposide	120 I.V.Sh.I. (100 for pts >60 yr old)	4,5,6	
LF	Leucovorin	200 I.V. bolus or 2-h inf	1–5	q. 28 d × 12
	5-Fluorouracil	400 I.V. bolus 1 h after starting LCV	1–5	
FCE	5-Fluorouracil	900/d I.V.C.I.	1–5	q. 21 d × 6
	Cisplatin	20 I.V. bolus with hydration, antiemetics	1–5	
	Etoposide	90 I.V.Sh.I	1,3,5	

Pancreatic Carcinoma (Advanced Unresectable, Recurrent or Metastatic)

Regimen	Drugs	Dose (mg/m^2) & admin. rte.	Days of treatment	Frequency & comments
FAM-S	5-Fluorouracil	600 I.V. bolus	1,8,29,36	q. 56 d × 6
	Doxorubicin (Adriamycin)	30 I.V. bolus	1 & 29	
	Mitomycin-C	10 I.V. bolus	1	
	Streptozotocin	400 I.V.Sh.I.	1,8,29,36	Monitor blood glucose
SMF	Streptozotocin	500 I.V.Sh.I.	1,8,29,36	q. 56 d
	Mitomycin-C	10 I.V. bolus		
	5-Fluorouracil	600 I.V. bolus	1,8,29,36	
SD	Streptozotocin	500 I.V.Sh.I.	1–5	q. 42 d
	Doxorubicin	50 I.V. bolus	1 & 22	

Apudomas of the G.I. Tract

Regimen	Drugs	Dose (mg/m^2) & admin. rte.	Days of treatment	Frequency & comments
SF	Streptozotocin	500 I.V.Sh.I.	1–5	q. 4–6 wk × 6 cyc
	5-Fluorouracil	400 I.V. bolus	1–5	
SA	Streptozotocin	500 I.V.Sh.I.	1–5	q. 6 wk × 6 cyc
	Doxorubicin (Adriamycin)	50 I.V. bolus	1 & 22	Monitor blood sugar

Colorectal Carcinoma

Regimen	Drugs	Dose (mg/m^2) & admin. rte.	Days of treatment	Frequency & comments
Advanced Metastatic Disease				
LF (weekly)	Leucovorin	500 I.V. 2-h inf	1 wk of 1–6	q. 8 wk × 2
	5-Fluorouracil	600 I.V. bolus 1 h after LCV is started	1 of wk 1–6	
LF (monthly)	Leucovorin	200 I.V. bolus	1–5	q. 4 wk × 12
	5-Fluorouracil	370–400 I.V. bolus 1 h after LCV is started	1–5	
MF	Mitomycin-C	10 I.V. bolus	1	q. 56 d × 6
	5-Fluourouracil	400 I.V. bolus	1–5 & 29–33	
F-INF	5-Fluorouracil	750 I.V. bolus	1–5, then on d 29	q. wk × 48
	Alpha interferon	9 million U s.c.	1,3,5	q. wk × 52
Surgical Adjuvant Therapy (for Stages C and B_3)				
F-Lev	5-Fluorouracil	450 I.V. bolus	1–5	
		then 450 I.V. bolus	1 each wk	× 48 doses
	Levamisole	150 (total dose/day) p.o.	1–3 q. 2 wk	× 26 doses

Carcinoma of the Rectum and Anus (Loco-Regional Disease)

MF + XRT Regimen

1. XRT to the lesion or residual tumor postoperatively; usually 5,000 cGy (200 cGy/d × 5 d/wk × 5 wk).
2. Mitomycin-C: 10 mg/m^2 I.V. bolus day 1 of XRT.
3. 5-Fluorouracil: 1,000 mg/m^2/d by I.V. C.I. × 5 in first and fourth week of XRT.

Carcinoma of the Biliary Tract (Loco-Regional Disease)

The same MF + XRT regimen as for carcinoma of the rectum and anus should be used. For metastatic disease, the LF and MF regimens used for advanced metastatic colorectal carcinoma should be used.

DOSE ADUSTMENTS—ALL REGIMENS USED IN G.I. MALIGNANCIES

1. For 5-fluorouracil, doxorubicin, mitomycin-C, and etoposide, the dose should be reduced to the degree of bone marrow suppression represented by the level of granulocyte and platelet count:

Granulocytes/μl	Platelets/μl	Dose administered
≥3,000	≥130,000	Full dose
2,000–2,990	100,000–129,900	75% of calc dose
1,500–1,990	75,000– 99,900	50% of calc dose
<1,500	<75,000	Hold therapy

2. For streptozotocin, the dose should be adjusted to serum glucose level (SGL):

SGL (fasting)	Dose administered
<120 mg/dl	Full dose
120–150 mg/dl	75% of calc dose
150–200 mg/dl	50% of calc dose
>200 mg	Administer only with insulin coverage

Malignancies of the Genitourinary System

Metastatic Testicular Cancer and other Germ Cell Tumors

Regimen	Drugs	Dose and admin. rte.	Days of treatment	Frequency & comments
PVB	Cisplatin (Platinol)	20 mg/m² I.V. 15 min with hydration NS inf + antiemetics	1–5	q. 3 wk × 3
	Vinblastine	0.15 mg/kg I.V. bolus (preferably 6 h before bleomycin)	1 & 2	A 4th cycle (without bleomycin) is given if no CR achieved
	Bleomycin	30 U I.V.Sh.I. D5%/½ NS after testing for allergy	1,8,15	
BEP	Cisplatin (Platinol)	20 mg/m² I.V. as above	1–5	q. 3 wk × 4 (omit bleomycin in last cyc)
	Etoposide	100 mg/m² I.V. 1-h NS inf	1–5	
	Bleomycin	30 U I.V.Sh.I. D5%/½ NS inf	1,8,15	
VAB-6 (induction)	Vinblastine	4 mg/m² I.V. bolus	1	q. 28 d × 3 (omit bleomycin in last cyc)
	Cyclophosphamide	600 mg/m² I.V. bolus	1	
	Actinomycin D	1 mg/m² I.V. bolus	1	
	Bleomycin	30 U I.V. bolus, then 20 U/m² by C.I.	1 1–3	
	Cisplatin	120 mg/m² I.V.Sh.I. NS c̄ mannitol, antiemetics	4	
VAB-6 (maintenance)	Vinblastine	4 mg/m² I.V. bolus	1	q. 3 wk × 24
	Actinomycin D	1 mg/m² I.V. bolus	1	
	Chlorambucil	4 mg/m²/d p.o.	1–14	
EP (induction)	Etoposide	100 mg/m² I.V.Sh.I. NS	1–5	q. 21 d × 6 (only for low-risk patients)
	Cisplatinum (Platinol)	20 mg/m² I.V. in 15-min NS inf with mannitol, antiemetics	1–5	
EP (maintenance)	Etoposide	200 mg/m²/d p.o.	1–5	q. 28 d × 24 (this adjuvant regimen recommended for high-risk pts)
Salvage Regimen				
VIMP	Vinblastine	0.22 mg/kg I.V. bolus	1	
	Ifosfamide	1.2 g/m² I.V.C.I.	1–5	q. 21 d × 4
	MESNA	120 mg I.V. bolus, then 1.2 g/m² I.V.C.I.	1–5	
	Cisplatin (Platinol)	20 mg/m² I.V.Sh.I.	1–5	
CVEB	Cisplatin	40 mg/m² I.V.Sh.I. with mannitol, hydration, antiemetics	1–5	q. 3 wk × 4 (D/C bleomycin after 90 U)
	Vinblastine	7.5 mg/m² I.V. bolus	1	
	Etoposide	100 mg/m² I.V.Sh.I.	1–5	
	Bleomycin	30 U I.V.Sh.I.	1 of wk 1–3	

Wilms' Tumor

Regimen	Drugs	Dose & admin. rte.	Days of treatment	Frequency & comments
AV	Actinomycin D	15 μg/kg I.V.Sh.I.	1–5 of wks 0,6,13,26—stg I plus in wks 40,49,58—stg II	In infants, dose is decreased to 7.5 μg/kg; this regimen is only for favorable histology stage I or II
	Vincristine	1.5 mg/m² (max 2 mg) I.V. bolus	1 of wk 1–10, then 1 of wk 13,26 for stg I; 1 of wk 15,24,33,42, 51,60 for stg II	
AVADR	Actinomycin D	15 μg/kg I.V.Sh.I.	1–5 of wk 0,6,13,26,39,52,65	For stage I or II (unfavorable histology) and for all stage III or IV cases
	Vincristine	1.5 mg/m² (max 2 mg) I.V. bolus	1 of wk 1–10; 1 & 5 of wk 13,26,39,52,65	
	Doxorubicin (Adriamycin)	20 mg/m² I.V. bolus	1,2,3 of wk 3,19,32,45,58	

Cancer of the Bladder and Urothelial Tract

Regimen	Drugs	Dose & admin. rte.	Days of treatment	Frequency & comments
M-VAC	Methotrexate	30 mg/m² I.V. bolus	1,15,22	q. 28 d × 4 (pts. who had prior XRT start doxorubicin at 15 mg/m²)
	Vinblastine	3 mg/m² I.V. bolus	2,15,22	
	Doxorubicin (Adriamycin)	30 mg/m² I.V. bolus	2	
	Cisplatin	70 mg/m² I.V.Sh.I. with mannitol, hydration, antiemetics	2	
CISCA	Cisplatin	70–100 mg/m² I.V.Sh.I. with mannitol, hydration, antiemetics	2	q. 21–28 d × 4
	Cyclophosphamide	650 mg/m² I.V.Sh.I.	1	
	Doxorubicin (Adriamycin)	50 mg/m² I.V. bolus	1	
CAP	Cyclophosphamide	400 mg/m² I.V.Sh.I. c̄ hydration	1	q. 21 d × 6
	Doxorubicin (Adriamycin)	40 mg/m² I.V. bolus	1	
	Cisplatin	60 mg/m² I.V. bolus c̄ mannitol, hydration, antiemetics	1	

Prostatic Cancer (Stage D_2—Hormonal Therapy Failure)

Regimen	Drugs	Dose & admin. rte.	Days of treatment	Frequency & comments
DMF	Doxorubicin	50 mg/m² I.V. bolus	1	q. 3 wk × 6
	Mitomycin-C	10 mg/m² I.V. bolus		
	5-Fluorouracil	750 mg/m² I.V. bolus	1 & 2	

DOSE ADJUSTMENTS—ALL REGIMENS USED IN THERAPY OF G.U. MALIGNANCIES

1. For vinblastine, etoposide, cyclosphosphamide, dactinomycin, doxorubicin, methotrexate, mitomycin-C, 5-fluorouracil, and chlorambucil, the dose should be adjusted to the degree of bone marrow suppression:

Granulocytes	Platelets	Dose administered
>3,000	>130,000	Full dose
2,000–2,990	100,000–129,900	75% of calc dose
1,500–1,990	75,000–99,000	50% of calc dose
<1,500	<75,000	Hold therapy

2. Dosage of cisplatin should be reduced in case of renal insufficiency:

Serum creat.	Creat. clearance	Dose administered
<1.5	>60 ml/min	Full dose
1.5–1.7	45–60 ml/min	50% of calc dose
>1.7	<45 ml/min	Hold therapy

3. For bleomycin, therapy should be discontinued if fibrotic changes appear on chest x-ray or if abnormalities of diffusion capacity or allergic reactions are manifested.

Gynecological Malignant Neoplasms

Metastatic Epithelial Ovarian Carcinoma

Regimen	Drugs	Dose & admin. rte.	Days of treatment	Frequency & comments
PAC (CAP)	Cisplatin (Platinol)	50 mg/m^2 I.V.Sh.I. c̄ mannitol, antiemetics, I.V. hydration	1	q. 3 wk × 8
	Doxorubicin (Adriamycin)	50 mg/m^2 I.V. bolus	1	
	Cyclophosphamide	500 mg/m^2 I.V.Sh.I.	1	
CP	Cyclophosphamide	1,000 mg/m^2 I.V.Sh.I.	1	q. 3 wk × 10
	Cisplatin (Platinol)	50–60 mg/m^2 I.V.Sh.I. c̄ mannitol, hydration, antiemetics	1	
CDC	Carboplatin	300 mg/m^2 I.V. bolus	1	q. 4 wk × 6
	Doxorubicin	40 mg/m^2 I.V. bolus	1	
	Cyclophosphamide	500 mg/m^2 I.V.Sh.I	1	
CC	Carboplatin	300 mg/m^2 I.V. bolus	1	q. 3–4 wk × 12
	Cyclophosphamide	1,000 mg/m^2 I.V.Sh.I.	1	
AP	Doxorubicin (Adriamycin)	50–60 mg/m^2 I.V. bolus	1	q. 3 wk × 6–8 cyc
	Cisplatin (Platinol)	50–60 mg/m^2 I.V.Sh.I. c̄ mannitol, hydration, antiemetics	1	
CHAP (or CHAD)	Cyclophosphamide	300–500 mg/m^2 I.V.Sh.I.	1	q. 4 wk × 6–8 cyc
	Hexamethylmelamine	150 mg/m^2 p.o.	1–7	
	Adriamycin	30–50 mg/m^2 I.V. bolus	1	
	Cisplatin (Platinol, *cis*-diamminedichloroplatinum)	50 mg/m^2 I.V.Sh.I. c̄ mannitol, antiemetics, I.V. hydration	1	

*Metastatic Germ Cell Ovarian Carcinoma**

Regimen	Drugs	Dose & admin. rte.	Days of treatment	Frequency & comments
VAC	Vincristine	1.2–1.5 mg/m^2 I.V. bolus (max 2 mg)	1	q. wk × 12
	Actinomycin D	0.3–0.4 mg/m^2 I.V.Sh.I.	1–5	q. 28 d
	Cyclosphosphamide	150 mg/m^2 I.V.Sh.I.	1–5	q. 28 d

*All regimens recommended for testicular germ cell carcinoma could also be used.

Gestational Trophoblastic Disease

Regimen	Drugs	Dose & admin. rte.	Days of treatment	Frequency & comments
DMC	Dactinomycin	0.30 mg/m^2 I.V.Sh.I.	1–5	q. 21 d × 8–10 cyc
	Methotrexate	11 mg/m^2 I.V. bolus	1–5	
	Cyclophosphamide	110 mg/m^2 I.V.Sh.I.	1–5	

Metastatic Carcinoma of the Uterine Corpus (Endometrial Carcinoma)

There is no standard regimen. The one given here is the most widely used.

Regimen	Drugs	Dose & admin. rte.	Days of treatment	Frequency & comments
AC(Meg)	Doxorubicin (Adriamycin)	60 mg/m² I.V. bolus		q. 31 d × 6–10 cyc
	Cisplatin	100 mg/m² Sh.I. NS c̄ mannitol, hydration, antiemetics	1	
	Megesterone acetate (Megace)	40 mg/ q.i.d. p.o.	1–21	If drug was not used while disease was progressing

Metastatic Squamous Cell Carcinoma of the Cervix, Vagina, and Vulva

There is no standard chemotherapy regimen for these neoplasms; however, some of the regimens used for the advanced squamous cell carcinoma of the head and neck can also be administered to these patients if they are not eligible for ongoing clinical trials. Other regimens that have been used with limited results are given below.

Regimen	Drugs	Dose & admin. rte.	Days of treatment	Frequency & comments
AM	Doxorubicin (Adriamycin)	50 mg/m² I.V. bolus	1	q. 3–4 wk × 6–8 cyc
	Methotrexate	20 mg/m² I.V. bolus	1 & 8	
BVMC	Bleomycin	7.5 U/m² I.V.C.I. NS	1–4 & 22–26	q. 56 d × 3
	Vincristine	0.5 mg I.V.C.I. NS or bolus (can be admixed c̄ BLM)	1–4 & 22–26	
	Mitomycin-C	20 mg/m² I.V. bolus	1	
BPVM	Bleomycin	5 U/m² I.V. 6-h or 24-h NS inf	1–5	q. 21 d × 6 (except D/C bleomycin after 4 cyc or if x-ray fibrosis develops)
	Cisplatin (Platinol)	25 mg/m² I.V. 6-h or 24-h NS inf (can be admixed c̄ BLM)	1–5	
	Vincristine	2 mg I.V. bolus	1	
	Methotrexate	200 mg/m² I.V. 1-h inf (with LCV 25 mg p.o. q. 6 h × 12 starting 24 h after start of MTX) *or*	1	
		40 mg/m² I.V. bolus	1	

NOTE: *Dose adjustments for gynecologic malignancies are similar to those recommended for gentourinary malignancies.*

Metastatic Carcinoma of the Breast

Regimen	Drugs	Dose & admin. rte.	Days of treatment	Frequency & comments
CMF	Cyclosphosphamide	100 mg/m^2/d p.o.	1–14	q. 28 d × 6 as adjuvant chemotherapy or as necessary for metastatic disease
	Methotrexate	40 mg/m^2 I.V. bolus (30 mg/m^2 for pts >60 yr old)	1 & 8	
	5-Fluorouracil	500 mg/m^2 I.V. bolus	1 & 8	
CMFP	Cyclophosphamide	100 mg/m^2 I.V. bolus	1–14	q. 28 d × 6+ cyc
	Methotrexate	40 mg/m^2 I.V. bolus (same medication as for CMF)	1 & 8	
	5-Fluourouracil	500 mg/m^2 I.V. bolus	1 & 8	
	Prednisone	40 mg/m^2 p.o., then taper over 5 d	1–14	In 1st 3 cyc only
CAF	Cyclophosphamide	600 mg/m^2 I.V. bolus	1	q. 21–28 d × 6–15 cyc
	Doxorubicin (Adriamycin)	45 mg/m^2 I.V. bolus	1	Substitute MTX 30 mg/m^2 for ADR when ADR cumulative dose of 450 mg/m^2 is reached
	5-Fluorouracil	600 mg/m^2 I.V. bolus	1	
CMFVP (Cooper's regimen)	Cyclophosphamide	2.0–2.5 mg/kg p.o.	1–270	q.d.
	Methotrexate	0.7 mg/kg/wk I.V.	1 then 1	q. wk × 8 q. 2 wk × 14
	5-Fluorouracil	12 mg/kg/wk I.V.	1 then 1	q. wk × 8 q. 2 wk × 14
	Vincristine	0.035 mg/kg/wk I.V.	1	q. wk × 5
	Prednisone	0.75 mg/kg/d p.o.	1–10, then taper over 40 d	q.d.
VATH	Vinblastine	4.5 mg/m^2 I.V.	1	q. 21 d × 6
	Doxorubicin (Adriamycin)	45 mg/m^2 I.V.	1	
	Thio-tepa	12 mg/m^2 I.V.	1	
	Fluoxymesterone (Halotestin)	30 mg p.o.	1–21	
IMF	Ifosfamide	1.5 g/m^2 I.V.	1 & 8	
	MESNA	300 mg/m^2 I.V. before & at 4 & 8 h after IFX	1 & 8	
	Methotrexate	40 mg/m^2 I.V.	1 & 8	
	5-Fluorouracil	600 mg/m^2 I.V.	1 & 8	
Salvage Regimens				
MiVb	Mitomycin-C	10 mg/m^2 I.V. push	1	q. 6 wk × 3–6 cyc
	Vinblastine	1.2 mg/m^2/d × 5 I.V.C.I.	1–5; 22–27	
MiVb	Mitomycin-C	10 mg/m^2 I.V. bolus	1	q. 6 wk × 3–6 cyc
	Vinblastine	6 mg/m^2 I.V. bolus	1 & 22	
MiVbC	Mitomycin-C	4 mg/m^2 I.V. bolus	1	q. 6 wk × 3–6 cyc
	Vinblastine	3 mg/m^2 I.V. bolus	1,15,29	
	Carmustine (BCNU)	50 mg/m^2 I.V.Sh.I.	1	
NoV	Mitoxantrone (Novantrone)	12 mg/m^2 I.V. bolus	1	q. 3 wk × 6 cyc
	Vincristine	1.5 mg/m^2 (max 2 mg) I.V. bolus	1	

Regimen	Drugs	Dose & admin. rte.	Days of treatment	Frequency & comments
NoVE	Mitoxantrone (Novantrone)	10 mg/m^2 I.V. bolus	1	q. 3–4 wk × 6
	Vincristine	1.5 mg/m^2 (max 2 mg) I.V. bolus	1	
	Etoposide	80 mg/m^2 I.V.Sh.I.	1–3	
		or		
		160 mg/m^2 p.o.	1–3	

DOSE ADJUSTMENTS—ALL REGIMENS FOR METASTATIC BREAST CARCINOMA

1. For bone marrow suppressing agents (e.g., methotrexate, 5-fluorouracil, doxorubicin, mitomycin-C, mitoxantrone, thio-tepa), dose reductions are related to the WBC and platelet count level:

Granulocytes/μl	Platelets/μl	Dose administered
>3,000	>130,000	Full dose
2,000–3,000	100,000–129,000	75% of calc dose
1,500–1,990	75,000–99,900	50% of calc dose
<1,500	<75,000	Hold therapy

2. For vincristine and vinblastine, the dose should be decreased by 50% if DTRs are decreased, and/or severe constipation persists or direct serum bilirubin is >2mg/dl. Medication should be withheld when DTRs are abolished or direct serum bilirubin is >2.5 mg/dl.

Medullary and Anaplastic Thyroid Carcinoma and Undifferentiated Nonsecretory Adrenal Cortical Carcinoma

Regimen	Drugs	Dose & admin. rte.	Days of treatment	Frequency & comments
DP	Doxorubicin (Adriamycin)	40–60 mg/m^2 I.V. bolus	1	q. 21 d × 6–10 cyc
	Cisplatin (Platinol)	60 mg/m^2 I.V. Sh.I. NS $\bar{c}$ mannitol, hydration, antiemetics	1	

Sarcomas

Soft-Tissue Sarcomas

Regimen	Drugs	Dose & admin. rte.	Days of treatment	Frequency & comments
Unresectable High-Grade or Metastatic in Adults				
ADIC	Doxorubicin (Adriamycin)	60 mg/m^2 I.V. bolus	1	q. 21 d × 6–8 cyc
	Dacarbazine (DIC)	250 mg/m^2 I.V.Sh.I.	1–5	
CYVADIC	Cyclophosphamide	500 mg/m^2 I.V. push	2	q. 28 d × 6–8 cyc
	Vincristine (Oncovin)	1.5 mg/m^2 (max 2 mg) I.V. push	1	
	Doxorubicin (Adriamycin)	50 mg/m^2 I.V. push	2	
	Dacarbazine (DIC)	250 mg/m^2 I.V.Sh.I.	1–5	
CYVADACT	Cyclophosphamide	500 mg/m^2 I.V. push	2	q. 28 d × 6–8 cyc
	Vincristine	1.5 mg/m^2 (max 2 mg) I.V. push	1	
	Doxorubicin (Adriamycin)	50 mg/m^2 I.V. push	2	
	Dactinomycin (Actinomycin-D)	0.3 mg/m^2/d (max 0.5 mg) I.V.Sh.I.	3–5	
ID	Ifosfamide	5 g/m^2 I.V.C.I. × 24 h	1	q. 21 d × 6–8 cyc
	Doxorubicin	40 mg/m^2 I.V. bolus	1	
	MESNA	1 g/m^2 I.V. bolus prior to ifosfamide, then 4 g/m^2 × 32 h	1	
MAID	MESNA	2,500 mg/m^2 I.V.C.I.	1–4	q. 3 wk for 6–8 cyc (Adriamycin & dacarbazine admin only through central I.V. line)
	Doxorubicin (Adriamycin)	20 mg/m^2 I.V.C.I.	1–3	
	Ifosfamide	2,500 mg/m^2 I.V.C.I. admixed with MESNA	1–3	
	Dacarbazine	300 mg/m^2 I.V.C.I. admixed with ADR	1–3	
Unresectable High-Grade or Metastatic in Children				
VAC	Vincristine	1.5 mg/m^2 (max 2 mg)	1	q. 21 d × 12
	Dactinomycin (Actinomycin-D)	0.3 mg/m^2/d (max 0.5 mg) I.V.Sh.I.	1–3	
	Cyclophosphamide	500 mg/m^2 I.V. push	2	
VADRC	Vincristine	1.5 mg/m^2 (max 2mg) I.V. bolus	1	q. 21 d × 12
	Doxorubicin (Adriamycin)	30 mg/m^2 I.V. bolus	1,2	
	Cyclophosphamide	500 mg/m^2 I.V.Sh.I.	2	
VADRC/VAC	VADRC regimen		wk. 0,3,12,20,28 3,6,44,52	
	VAC regimen		wk 6,9,16,24,32,40,48; after wk 52, q. 4 wk. for another yr	
VAC (protracted)	Vincristine	2 mg/m^2 (max 2 mg)	1 of wk 1–12	
	Dactinomycin (Actinomycin D)	0.015 mg/kg (max 0.5 mg) I.V.Sh.I.	1–5	q. 3 mo × 6
	Cyclophosphamide	2.5 mg/kg/d p.o.		q.d. × 2 yr

Osteosarcomas (Metastatic or Residual Disease)

Regimen	Drugs	Dose & admin. rte.	Days of treatment	Frequency & comments
HDMTX/VCR	Methotrexate (high-dose)	100–750 mg/kg (children) 8–12 g/m² (adults) I.V. inf 4–6 h preceded by urine alkalization & I.V. hydration		q. 14–21 d × 12 (monitor serum MTX level)
	Leucovorin	15 mg p.o. (start 6–12 h after MTX is started; then q. 6 h × 12)	1–3	
	Vincristine	1.4 mg/m² (max 2 mg) I.V. bolus	1	
HDMTX/ADR	Methotrexate (high-dose)	100–750 mg/kg (children) 8–12 g/m² (adults) I.V. inf over 4 h	1	q. 28 d × 6 with same precautions for I.V. hydration, urine alkalinization, and serum MTX monitoring
	Leucovorin	15 mg p.o. (start 2 h after MTX) q. 6 h × 12	1–3	
	Doxorubicin (Adriamycin)	0.80 mg/kg/d (children) I.V. bolus 45 mg/m²/day (adults) I.V. bolus	15–17 15,16	
HDMTX/A/C	Methotrexate (high-dose)	100–750 mg/kg (children) 1–7 g/m² (adults) I.V. inf over 4 h	1	q. 28 d × 6 (same precautions as above)
	Leucovorin	15 mg p.o. (start 2 h after MTX) q. 6 h × 12	1–3	
	Doxorubicin (Adriamycin)	50 mg/m² I.V. bolus	15	
	Cyclosphosphamide	500 mg/m² I.V. bolus	15	
BCD	Bleomycin	12 U/m² I.V.Sh.I.	1 & 2	q. 14 d × 5, then continue s̄ BLM
	Cyclosphosphamide	600 mg/m² I.V.Sh.I.	1	
	Dactinomycin (Actinomycin D)	0.45 mg/m² I.V.Sh.I.	1 & 2	

*Osteosarcomas—Adjuvant Therapy**

Regimen	Drugs	Dose & admin. rte.	Days/weeks of treatment	Frequency & comments
Preoperative Induction Phase (Neoadjuvant Therapy)				
	Surgery:			
	Amputation		1 of 4th wk	
	Endoprosthesis		1 of 16th wk	
MV/BCD/A	Methotrexate (high-dose)	8–12 g/m² I.V. inf 1,000 U D5%/½ NS over 4 h (in children max 450 mg/kg)	1 of wk 1,2, 3,4,9,10,14,15	
	Leucovorin	25 mg p.o. q. 6 h × 12 (start 6 h after MTX inf onset)	1,2,3, of wk 1–4,9,10,14,15	
	Vincristine	1.4 mg/m² (max 2 mg) before MTX	1 of wk 1–4,9,10,14,15	
	Bleomycin	12 U/m² I.V.Sh.I.	1 of 6th wk	
	Cyclophosphamide	600 mg/m² I.V.	1 of 6th wk	
	Dactinomycin (Actinomycin D)	0.60 mg/m² I.V.Sh.I.	1 of 6th wk	
	Doxorubicin (Adriamycin)	30 mg/m² I.V. bolus × 3 d	1 of 11th wk	

*Pre- and postoperation—T-10 MSKCC

Regimen	Drugs	Dose & admin. rte.	Days/weeks of treatment	Frequency & comments
Postoperative Adjuvant Therapy				
1. For Poor Responders to Preoperative Chemotherapy:				
AC/BCD	Doxorubicin (Adriamycin)	30 mg/m^2 I.V. bolus × 2 d	1 of 1st & 4th wk	q. 10 wk × 3
	Cisplatin	120 mg/m^2 I.V. in NS 250 cc inf c̄ mannitol, antiemetics	1 of 1st & 4th wk	
	Bleomycin	12 U/m^2 I.V.Sh.I.	1 of 7th wk	
	Cyclophosphamide	600 mg/m^2 I.V.	1 of 7th wk	
	Dactinomycin	0.60 mg/m^2 I.V.Sh.I.	1 of 7th wk	
2. For Patients with Good Response to Preoperative Chemotherapy:				
MVA	Methotrexate (high-dose)	8–12 g/m^2 I.V. in 1,000 cc D5%/½ NS over 4 h	1 of wk 4,5,9,10	q. 12 wk q. 12 wk
	Leucovorin	25 mg p.o. q. 6 h × 12 (starting 6 h after MTX inf onset)		
	Vincristine	1.4 mg/m^2 (max 2 mg) I.V.	1 of wk 4,5,9,10	
	Doxorubicin (Adriamycin)	30 mg/m^2 × 3 d I.V.	1 of 6th wk	

Neuroblastoma (Stages III and IV)

Regimen	Drugs	Dose & admin. rte.	Days of treatment	Frequency & comments
CVD	Cyclophosphamide	750 mg/m^2 I.V.Sh.I.	1	q. 21 d × 6–10 cyc
	Vincristine	1.5 mg/m^2 (max 2 mg) I.V. bolus	5	
	Dacarbazine	250 mg/m^2 I.V.Sh.I.	1–5	
CA	Cyclophosphamide	150 mg/m^2/d p.o.	1–7	q. 21–28 d × 6–10 cyc
	Doxorubicin (Adriamycin)	35 mg/m^2 I.V. bolus	8	

Malignant Melanoma

Regimen	Drugs	Dose & admin. rte.	Days of treatment	Frequency & comments
BHD	Carmustine (BCNU)	100–150 mg/m^2 I.V.Sh.I.	1	q 6 wk × 6
	Hydroxyurea	1,480 mg/m^2/d p.o.	1–5; 22–26	
	Dacarbazine	100–150 mg/m^2 I.V.Sh.I.	1–5; 22,26	
D-Act	Dacarbazine	750 mg/m^2 I.V.Sh.I.	1	q. 4 wk × 6
	Dactinomycin (Actinomycin D)	1 mg/m^2 I.V.Sh.I.	1	
VBD	Vinblastine	6 mg/m^2 I.V. bolus	1 & 2	q. 28 d × 4–6 cyc
	Bleomycin	15 U/m^2/d I.V.C.I.	1–5	
	Cis-diamminedichloroplatinum (Platinol)	50 mg/m^2 I.V.Sh.I. $\bar{c}$ hydration, mannitol, antiemetics	5	
VDP	Vinblastine	5 mg/m^2 I.V. bolus	1 & 2	q. 21–28 d × 4–6 cyc
	Dacarbazine	150 mg/m^2 I.V.Sh.I.	1–5	
	Cisplatin (Platinol)	75 mg/m^2 I.V.Sh.I. $\bar{c}$ hydration, mannitol, antiemetics	5	
DBTC	Dacarbazine	220 mg/m^2/d I.V.Sh.I.	1–3; 22–24	q 6 wk × 4
	Carmustine (BCNU)	150 mg/m^2 I.V.Sh.I.	1	
	Tamoxifen	10 mg p.o. b.i.d.	daily	
	Cisplatin	25 mg/m^2/d I.V.Sh.I.	1–3; 22–24	
CBC	Lomustine (CCNU)	80 mg/m^2 p.o.	1	q 6 wk × 6
	Bleomycin	15 U/m^2/d I.V.Sh.I.	3–7	
	Cisplatin	40 mg/m^2/d I.V.Sh.I.	8	
BELD	Bleomycin	15 mg s.c.	1–4	q 4–6 wk × 6
	Vindesine (Eldisine)	3 mg/m^2 I.V.	1 & 5	
	Lomustine	80 mg/m^2 p.o.	1	
	Dacarbazine	200 mg/m^2 I.V.Sh.I.	1–5	
DVC	Dacarbazine	250 mg/m^2 I.V.Sh.I.	1–5	q 4–6 wk × 6
	Vindesine	3 mg/m^2 I.V. bolus	1	
	Cisplatin	100 mg/m^2 in 500 ml NS $\bar{c}$ antiemetics & heavy hydration	1	
POC	Procarbazine	100 mg/m^2 (max 150 mg) p.o.	1–10	q. 4–6 wk × 6
	Vincristine (Oncovin)	1.4 mg/m^2 (max 2 mg) I.V. bolus	1 & 8	
	Lomustine (CCNU)	150 mg/m^2 (max 200 mg) p.o.	1	

Supportive Therapy

Antiemetic Therapy: Current Dosage and Scheduling Recommendations

Class/drug	Recommended dosage and schedule	Comments
Phenothiazenes		
Prochlorperazine	5–10 mg I.V. or orally q. 4–6 h; 25 mg q. 6 h	Diphenhydramine 25–50 mg may be given with each dose
Perphenazine	Loading dose of 2–5 mg over 60 min; then 2–4 mg I.V. or orally q. 4 h (or 0.5 mg/h C.I.)	Diphenhydramine 25–50 mg may be given with each dose
Thiethylperazine	10 mg q. 4–6 h	Available in oral, I.M., and rectal forms
Benzquinamides		
Benzquinamide	50 mg q. 4 h or 25 mg q. 2–4 h I.M.	
Trimethobenzamide	250 mg p.o. or 200 mg supp. q. 4 h	
Butyrophenones		
Haloperidol	0.5–1 mg orally or I.M. q. 8 h	
Droperidol	Loading dose of 10 mg I.V.; then 2 mg/h by C.I. during chemotherapy admin.	
Substituted benzamides		
Metoclopramide	1–2 mg/kg I.V. 30 min before chemotherapy and repeated every 2 h for 2 doses, then every 3 h for 3 doses	0.75 mg/kg/dose may be given for less emetogenic regimens. Diphenhydramine 50 mg may be given with the first dose
Corticosteroids		
Dexamethasone	8–10 mg I.V. q. 6 h for 4 doses	
Cannabinoids		
Tetrahydro-cannabinol	10 mg orally (max 15 mg) 4–5 h before chemotherapy; then q. 4 h during chemotherapy admin.	
Hypnotics and sedatives		
Lorazepam	1.5–2 mg/kg I.V. or sublingually (max 4 mg) q. 12 h	
$5HT_3$ receptor antagonists		
Ondansetron (GR38032F)	0.15 mg/kg I.V. piggyback in 50 ml NS over 15 min before chemotherapy, then q 3–4 hr × 2 doses or 1 mg/hr × 24 hr C.I. if needed	Occasional constipation and headaches may occur

Narcotic Analgesics Widely Used for Severe Pain

Name	Route	Dose (mg)	Peak (h)	Duration (h)	Plasma half-life (h)	Comments
Morphinelike agonists						
Morphine	I.M.	10	0.5–1	4–6	2–3.5	Standard of comparison for narcotic-type analgesics
	p.o.	60	1.5–2	4–7		
Morphine (long-acting) (MS Contin or Roxanol)	p.o.	60	6	8–12		
Codeine	I.M.	130	0.5–1	4–6	3	Like morphine; excellent oral potency
	p.o.	200				
Hydromorphone (Dilaudid)	I.M.	1.5	0.5–1	4–5	2–3	
	p.o.	7.5	1.5–2	4–7		
Levorphanol (Levo-Dromoran)	I.M.	2	0.5–1	4–6	12–16	
	p.o.	4	1.5–2	4–7		
Meperidine (Demerol)	I.M.	75	0.5–1	4–5	3–4	Slightly shorter acting; poor oral potency
	p.o.	300	1.2	4–6		
Methadone (Dolophine)	I.M.	10	0.5–1	4–6	15–30	Good oral potency
	p.o.	20	1.5–2	4–7		
Oxycodone	p.o.	30	1	4–6	na	Available only (5-mg doses) in combination with acetaminophen or aspirin
Oxymorphone	I.M.	1	0.5–1	4–6	na	
Mixed agonist/antagonists						
Pentazocine	I.M.	60	0.5–1	4–6	2–3	Mixed agonist/antagonist; less abuse liability than morphine; included in schedule IV of Controlled Substances Act
	p.o.	180	1.5–2	4–7		
Butorphanol	I.M.	2	0.5–1	4–6	2.5–3.5	
Nalbuphine	I.M.	10	0.5–1	4–6	5	
Partial agonists						
Buprenorphine (Buprenex)	I.M.	0.4	0.5–1	4–6	na	Partial agonist of the morphine type; less abuse liability than morphine; does not produce psychotomimetic effects
	s.c.	0.8	2–3	5–6		

Current Antidepressant Medications

Generic name	Trade names (U.S.)	Dose range/day	Plasma levels (ng/ml)
Heterocyclics			
Amitriptyline HCl	Elavil, Etraphon Endep, Limbitrol Triavil	175–300	100–250
Amoxapine HCl	Asendin	100–600	–
Desipramine HCl	Norpramin, Pertofrane	100–300	100–300
Doxepin HCl	Adapin, Sinequan	25–300	100–200
Fluoxetine HCl	Prozac	20–80	–
Imipramine HCl	Tofranil, Janimine	30–300	150–300
Maprotiline HCl	Ludiomil	225–300	200–500
Nortriptyline HCl	Aventyl, Pamelor	20–150	50–150
Protriptyline HCl	Vivactyl	25–300	100–200
Trimipramine maleate	Surmontil	25–300	–
Other classes			
Alprazolam	Xanax	1.5–4.5	–
Trazodone HCl	Desyrel	50–600	–

Supportive Treatment Orders for High-Dose Chemotherapy

SUPPORTIVE TREATMENT DURING INTERMEDIATE AND HIGH-DOSE THERAPY (>20 MG/M^2/DOSE) WITH CISPLATIN

Treatment should not be instituted if patient has creatinine clearance ≤60 ml/24 hr or a platelet count of ≤75,000/μl.

The following orders are recommended for the first administration of cisplatin (DDP) dissolved in 250 cc NS and infused (usually over 1-hr period). They can be adjusted for the second cycle in accordance with the intensity of the side effects or lack thereof generated by the first administration.

1. Cisplatin (________)* I.V. in 250 cc NS over 1–2 hr.

2. Oral hydration during the 16 hr preceding DDP administration (at least 2,000 ml liquids).

3. Mannitol 12.5 g I.V. bolus before DDP or added to the DDP infusion.

4. Prochlorperazine 10 mg I.V. piggyback before DDP, then q. 6 hr I.V. piggyback or p.o. × 8.

5. Dexamethasone 10 mg I.V. PB before DDP, then q. 6 hr I.V. PB or p.o. × 4.

6. Ranetidine 150 mg p.o. b.i.d. × 3 days.

7. Lorazepam 1 mg p.o. b.i.d. × 3 days.

8. Metoclopromide 75–100 mg I.V. piggyback before DDP, then q. 2 hr × 2.

9. Diphenhydramine hydrochloride 25 mg I.V. piggyback before first and third dose of metoclopromide.

10. I.V. hydration: 1,000 ml D5%/½ NS with KCl 20 mEq over 4–6 hr following DDP administration.

11. Magnesium oxide 400 mg or magnesium gluconate 500 mg p.o. t.i.d. following DDP × 7 days.

12. Dronabinol 5 mg p.o. q. 4 hr × 6 doses can be added to previous orders if patient still has had nausea and vomiting (first dose 3 hr before chemotherapy).

---

*Space is left for addition of the indicated dose of DDP in various regimens.

SUPPORTIVE TREATMENT DURING INTERMEDIATE AND HIGH-DOSE THERAPY (>100 MG/M²/DOSE) WITH METHOTREXATE (MTX)

Treatment should not be instituted if patient has creatinine clearance of ≤60 mg/24 hr, platelet count of ≤100,000/μl, granulocyte count of ≤3000/μl, and/or urine pH of ≤6.

The following orders are recommended for the first MTX infusion. They can be adjusted for the second cycle in accordance with the intensity of side effects or lack thereof generated by the first administration.

1. MTX (preservative free) (________)* mg I.V. in D 5%/½ NS at a concentration of 2 mg/ml up to maximum dilution of 1,000 ml to be administered at a rate of 250 cc/hr.

2. Oral hydration during the 16 hr preceding the MTX administration (at least 2,000 ml liquids) and continuing for 48 hr after MTX (3,000 ml/24 hr).

3. Sodium bicarbonate 500–1,000 mg p.o. t.i.d. 24 hr prior and 72 hr after MTX administration (to keep urine pH > 6 < 7.5). If patient cannot take p.o. medication it can be administered I.V.

4. Prochlorperazine 10 mg I.V. piggyback before MTX then p.o. q.i.d. × 2 days.

5. Leucovorin:
   —15 mg p.o. starting 24 hr after start of MTX infusion of maximum 1,000 mg/m², then q. 6 hr × 7 or until serum MTX level is $<10^{-11}$ mEq/L.
   —25 mg I.V. in 100 ml D5%/½ NS 6 hr after starting MTX dose of >1 g/m², then p.o. q. 6 hr × 11 or until serum MTX level is $<10^{-11}$ mEq/L.

*Space is left for addition of the indicated dose of MTX in various regimens.

SUPPORTIVE TREATMENT DURING HIGH-DOSE I.V. THERAPY (>1 G/M²/DOSE) WITH CYTARABINE (ARA-C)

The following orders are recommended for administration of high-dose ara-C:

1. Cytosine arabinoside (________)* mg I.V. in 500 ml D5%/½ NS over 3 hr, usually q. 12 hr × 3–7 days.

2. Steroid ophthalmic solution (Cortisporin) 2 drops each eye q. 6 hr × 10 days.

3. Prochlorperazine 10 mg I.V. piggyback q. 6–8 hr throughout duration of ara-C infusion.

4. Lorazepam p.o. b.i.d. × 7–10 days.

5. I.V. hydration with D5%/½ NS 84–126 cc/126 cc/hr as tolerated.

6. Add KCl 40–80 mEq/L of fluids as needed.

*Space is left for addition of the indicated dose of ara-C in various regimens.

Dose Adjustments of Chemotherapy Drugs Related to Abnormalities of Various Systems and Organs

The following composite table lists the adjustments that should be made in the calculated dosage of various chemotherapy agents in relation to various tissue or organ abnormalities that develop and are still present at the time the drug is scheduled to be administered again. Dose reductions recommended should be regarded only as general guidelines to be corroborated with other factors such as previous treatment with XRT at sites containing a significant proportion of body's bone marrow; nutritional status; nadir of blood count; and age if over 75. Various combination regimens may have specific dose attenuation requirements derived from long-term experience with these regimens.

It is important to mention that it is generally advisable before reducing the dose of various drugs to postpone the administration of the whole combination regimen for 1 wk (maximum 2) when the dose reduction may not be necessary; this in view of the fact that maintaining the intensity of the dose of most chemotherapeutic regimens has been found to be the most important factor contributing to their full efficacy. It is also likely that these recommendations, especially those concerning the adjustments due to bone marrow suppression, may need to be drastically changed in the future, when the concomitant administration of colony-stimulating factors with cytotoxic agents could become common practice.

Drug	Platelet counts ($10^{-3}/\mu l$)			Granulocyte counts ($10^{-3}/\mu l$)			Creatinine clearance (ml/min)		Direct bilirubin (mg/dl)			DTRs		Comments
	<130 ≥100	<100 ≥75	<75	<3.0 ≥2.0	<2.0 ≥1.5	<1.5	<60 ≥45	<45	>1.2 ≤1.5	>1.5 ≤2.5	>2.5	±	Absent	
m-AMSA	—	—	—	—	—	—	—	—	—	50	75	—	—	
Bleomycin	—	—	—	—	—	—	—	50	—	—	—	—	—	D/C† in case of pulmon. fibrosis on x-ray or ↓ pulmon. diffus. cap.
Carmustine (BCNU)	25*	50	hold	25	50	hold	—	—	—	—	—	—	—	
Cisplatin	—	25	50	—	—	—	50**	hold	—	—	—	—	—	D/C if hearing loss (by audiometry) develops; give Mg suppl if serum Mg <1.5 mEq/L or <2 mg/dl
Cyclophosphamide	25	50	hold	25	50	hold	—	50	—	—	—	—	—	Hold if proper fluid intake cannot be provided; D/C in case of cystitis
Cytarabine	25	50	hold	25	50	hold	—	—	—	—	—	—	—	Dose reductions do not apply to treatment of leukemia
Dacarbazine	25	50	hold	25	50	hold	—	—	—	—	—	—	—	
Dactinomycin	25	50	hold	25	50	hold	—	—	—	—	—	—	—	
Daunorubicin	25	50	hold	25	50	hold	—	—	25	50	75	—	—	Dose reductions do not apply for acute leukemias; D/C if LVEF§ <40%
Doxorubicin	25	50	hold	25	50	hold	—	—	25	50	75	—	—	
Etoposide	25	50	hold	25	50	hold	—	—	25	50	75			
Fludarabine	25	50	hold	25	50	hold	—	—	—	—	—	—	—	
Fluorouracil	25	50	hold	25	50	hold	—	25	—	—	—	—	—	
Hexamethylmelamine	25	50	hold	25	50	hold	—	—	—	—	—	—	—	
Hydroxyurea	25	50	hold	25	50	hold	—	—	—	—	—	—	—	In CML dose reductions, follow a specific schedule
Lomustine (CCNU)	25	50	hold	25	50	hold	—	—	—	—	—	—	—	
Mechlorethamine	25	50	hold	25	50	hold	—	—	—	—	—	—	—	
Melphalan														
Mecaptopurine														

Drug	Platelet counts ($10^{-3}/\mu l$)			Granulocyte counts ($10^{-3}/\mu l$)			Creatinine clearance (ml/min)		Direct bilirubin (mg/dl)			DTRs		Comments
	<130 ≥100	<100 ≥75	<75	<3.0 ≥2.0	<2.0 ≥1.5	<1.5	<60 ≥45	<45	>1.2 ≤1.5	>1.5 ≤2.5	>2.5	±	Absent	
Methotrexate	25	50	hold	25	50	hold	50	hold	—	50	hold	—	—	Hold if liver enzymes deteriorate, if proper hydration is not possible, or if urine pH is not >6; reduce dose or hold if 3rd space fluid is present
Mitomycin-C	25	50	hold	25	50	hold	—	50	—	—	—	—	—	D/C if fibrosis develops on chest x-ray or any unexplained deterioration of renal function or hemolysis occurs
Mitoxantrone	25	50	hold	25	50	hold	—	—	25	50	75	—	—	D/C in case of cardiac arrhythmia
Procarbazine	25	50	hold	25	50	hold	—	—	—	—	—	—	—	
Streptozotocin	—	—	—	—	—	—	—	50	—	—	—	—	—	
Thioguanine	25	50	hold	25	50	hold	—	—	—	—	—	—	—	
Triethylene-thiophospheramide	25	50	hold	25	50	hold	—	—	—	—	—	—	—	
Vinblastine	—	25	hold	25	50	hold	—	—	25	50	75	50	hold	D/C in case of paralytic ileus
Vincristine	—	—	—	—	25	hold	—	—	25	50	75	50	hold	

*Dose reduction given in % to be subtracted from original calculated dose

**Cisplatin dose adjusted only during course of ongoing treatment; no patient should initially receive drug if creatinine clearance is <60 ml/min

†Discontinue

§LVEF = left ventricular ejection fraction

Table A-1. Abbreviations and Symbols Used in this Appendix

Note: In specifying the days of a treatment cycle on which a drug is administered, a hyphen between 2 numbers indicates that drug is to be administered daily during the period of time defined by the 2 numbers, inclusive of the second number. An ampersand (&) between 2 numbers indicates that the drug is to be administered on the specified days of the treatment cycle.

ADR	doxorubicin
b.i.d.	twice a day
$\bar{c}$	with
calc dose	calculated dose
CALGB	Cancer and Acute Leukemia Group B
cGy	centigray (1 cGy = 1 rad)
CR	complete response
CSF	cerebrospinal fluid
cyc	cycle
D5%/½ NS	5% dextrose/half normal saline solution
D5%/W	5% dextrose/water solution
D/C	discontinue
DDP	cisplatin
DTR	deep tendon reflex
d	day
h	hour
inf	infusion
I.M.	intramuscular
I.V.C.I.	intravenous continuous infusion
I.V.Sh.I.	intravenous short infusion
IFX	ifosfamide
i.thec.	intrathecally
IU	international unit
kg	kilogram
LCV	leucovorin
max	maximum
m^2	meter squared
MSKCC	Memorial Sloan-Kettering Cancer Center
Mg	magnesium
mg	milligram
MTX	methotrexate
mo	month
NCI	National Cancer Insitute
ng	nanogram (= millimicrogram)
NS	normal saline solution
p.o.	orally
q.	every
q.d.	once daily
q. 5 d, etc.	every 5 days, etc.
q. 2 wk, etc.	every 2 weeks, etc.
q. 2 d × 6, etc.	every 2 days until 6 doses have been given, etc.
$\bar{s}$	without
s.c.	subcutaneous(ly)
supp. meas.	supportive measures
t.i.d.	3 times a day
U	unit
WBC	white blood cell (count)
wk	week
XRT	radiation therapy
yr	year
/	per
>	more than
<	less than

PLEASE NOTE:

Precept Press, Inc.
160 E. Illinois Street
Chicago, IL 60611

COMBINATION CHEMOTHERAPY AND SUPPORTIVE THERAPY IN NEOPLASTIC DISEASES

A Compendium of
Regimens and Schedules
of Administration from
Neoplastic Diseases: Fundamentals of Clinical Oncology

Edited by
C. Julian Rosenthal, M.D., F.A.C.P.

PLEASE NOTE:

Precept Press, Inc.
160 E. Illinois Street
Chicago, IL 60611

Contents